The Holistic (

Uncovering Secrets Big Pharma Prefers to keep hidden.

Natural Herbal Solutions for Everyday Ailments

"For every disease known to mankind, there is a plant somewhere in the world that holds the cure."

The Herbs are for the healing of the nations. Certified and licensed Herbalist.

FOR PARENTS, HEALTH WORKERS, STUDENTS AND TRADITIONAL DOCTORS

Please take your time reading this instruction manual and absorb its contents fully.

Benson Stephen

For more information and support contact:
herbalifenaturescure@gmail.com

Disclaimer Notice:

Please note that this document is intended for educational and informational purposes only. Every effort has been made to ensure the information is as accurate, current, reliable, and comprehensive as possible. However, the content in this book is derived from various natural herbal sources. If you do not fully understand any of the strategies mentioned, please consult us via email for further clarification before using them.

By using this information, whether or not it contains errors or inaccuracies, you acknowledge that the author is not liable for any direct or indirect damages resulting from your reliance on the content provided.

ISBN: 978-1-300-93126-3

Author: Benson Stephen

Book Title: The Holistic Guide to Wellness: Uncovering Secrets Big Pharma Prefers to Keep Hidden - Natural Herbal Solutions for Everyday Ailments

2

For more information and support contact:
herbalifenaturescure@gmail.com

Acknowledgment

Thank you from the bottom of my heart to everyone who has helped make **The Holistic Guide to Wellness** a reality. Devotion to the restorative power of nature, together with years of study and personal discovery, has culminated in this book. Everyone who had faith in the power of natural healing and pushed me to investigate herbal therapies has my undying gratitude.

To the traditional healers and herbalists whose insights formed the bedrock of this work, I offer my deepest gratitude. The foundation for many of the cures presented here may be found in their time-honored practices for treating obesity, cancer, fever, and other diseases.

Our deepest gratitude goes out to those who have contributed wisdom on the many facets of human health, especially as it pertains to men's innate sexual drive, women's natural lubrication, and men's strong libido. By bringing together contemporary research and traditional traditions, your contributions have made this book an all-inclusive resource for holistic health.

Last but not least, **The Holistic Guide to Wellness** is for those readers who are looking to build a stronger bond between their well-being and the natural world. With any luck, this book will provide you the tools you need to live a full, balanced life by embracing the restorative power of nature.

Incredibly grateful to everyone who has played a role in our adventure. We may keep on healing and thriving by utilizing the natural cures that are all around us if we work together.

For more information and support contact:
herbalifenaturescure@gmail.com

TABLE OF CONTENTS

For more information and support contact:
herbalifenaturescure@gmail.com

For more information and support contact:
herbalifenaturescure@gmail.com

Preface

Welcome to The Holistic Guide to Wellness: Herbal Remedies for Common Ailments This book is a helpful resource for anyone seeking alternative therapies for many health concerns. Herbal medicine, based on natural cures, has been fundamental to therapeutic techniques throughout various cultures and historical eras. Currently, as an increasing number of individuals acknowledge the advantages of holistic health, this understanding is more pertinent than ever.

This book will examine efficacious herbal teas and remedies for problems like obesity, fever, diminished libido in males, and natural lubrication in women, Kidney stones, Diabete, and others. Phytotherapeutic qualities can enhance immune function, promote general well-being, and reestablish bodily equilibrium. These natural medicines provide an alternative to traditional drugs by enhancing energy and immunity.

Nonetheless, although herbal remedies might be advantageous, it is crucial to recognize that they may not be effective for all individuals. Individual health, allergies, and lifestyle variations might influence the effectiveness of natural therapies. Consequently, it is important to seek the counsel of a healthcare expert prior to integrating any herbal beverages or medicines into your regimen to ascertain their safety and appropriateness.

This book serves as a guide to the therapeutic benefits of nature, while promoting respect for the individual requirements of your body. Seize this opportunity to explore the therapeutic potential of local flora and their role in enhancing your health and well-being.

For more information and support contact:
herbalifenaturescure@gmail.com

CHAPTER ONE

COCONUT PEELS (HUSK) REMEDIES

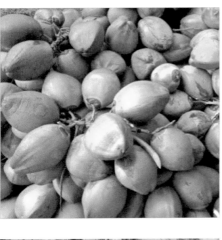
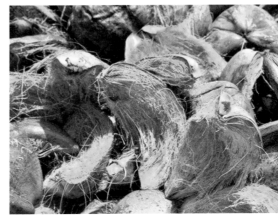
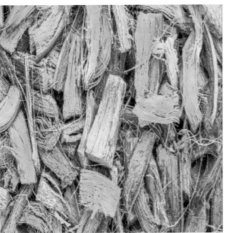
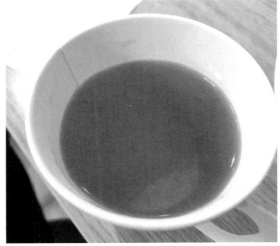

For more information and support contact:
herbalifenaturescure@gmail.com

Coconut Peels (Husks): A Natural Remedy for Various Ailments

Don't throw away coconut peels (husks); they hold potential as an effective treatment for several health conditions, including:

🌿 Kidney stones

🌿 Candidiasis (yeast infections)

🌿 Gonorrhea

🌿 Hypertension (high blood pressure)

🌿 Diabetes

🌿 Stomach ulcers

🌿 Diarrhea

🌿 Urinary tract infections (UTIs)

How to Use:

Preparation: Dry the coconut peels thoroughly.

Boiling: Boil the dried peels in water for 15 minutes.

Consumption: Strain and drink the liquid as tea twice daily.

Nature offers healing through these simple remedies.

For further verification, consult research on this topic through platforms like ResearchGate or scientific journals.

For more information and support contact:
herbalifenaturescure@gmail.com

CHAPTER TWO

BOOST YOUR PASSION: TRIED-AND-TRUE METHODS FOR INCREASING A MAN'S NATURAL SEXUAL DESIRE

BITTER KOLA, AND GINGER REMEDY

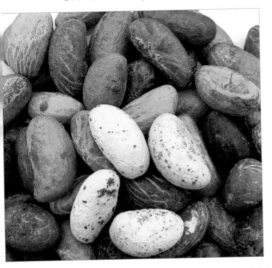

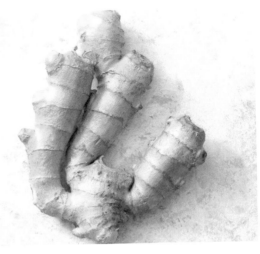

For more information and support contact:
herbalifenaturescure@gmail.com

Gentlemen, No Need to Worry If You Struggle with Stamina

If you're finding it difficult to last beyond two minutes during intimacy, don't worry—there's a natural remedy you can try.

Instructions for Preparation:

Ingredients:

- ❖ Chop five pieces of bitter kola.

- ❖ Slice one piece of ginger into small pieces.

Boiling:

- ❖ Combine the bitter kola and ginger in water and bring to a boil.

Usage:

- ❖ Drink one cup of this herbal tea 30 minutes before sexual activity.

This natural solution may help enhance your stamina, and soon enough, you'll feel like you've earned the "captain's band" in the bedroom!

For more information and support contact:
herbalifenaturescure@gmail.com

UNLOCK ENHANCED PASSION: UNDERSTANDING AND EMBRACING HIGH LIBIDO AND NATURAL LUBRICATION IN WOMEN

GORANTULA REMEDY

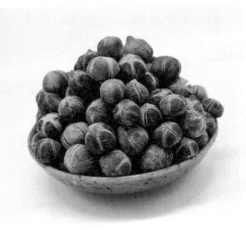

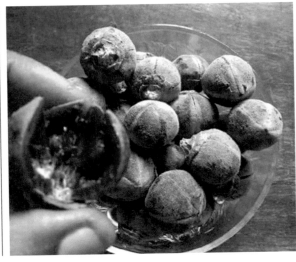

For more information and support contact:
herbalifenaturescure@gmail.com

Gorantula: A Natural Aid for Female Arousal and Lubrication

Gorantula is known to naturally increase female arousal and enhance lubrication.

How to Use:

Recommendation:

❖ Offer her three Gorantula fruits daily to enjoy their sweet nectar.

Benefits:

❖ Enhanced natural lubrication

❖ Increased libido

❖ Reduced risk of vaginal infections

This simple, natural remedy promotes overall reproductive health and well-being. Nature offers the cure!

For more information and support contact:
herbalifenaturescure@gmail.com

CHAPTER FOUR

CASSAVA LEAVES AND GINGER REMEDIES

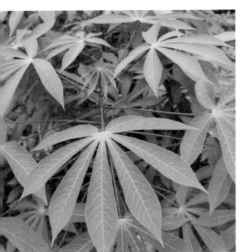

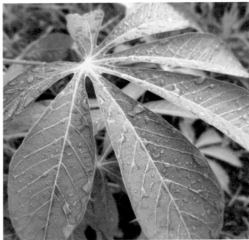

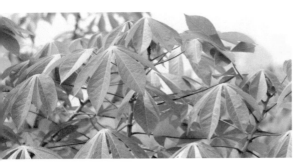

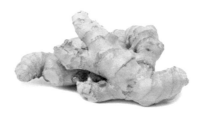

For more information and support contact:
herbalifenaturescure@gmail.com

Cassava Leaves: A Natural Remedy for Various Ailments

Cassava leaves offer powerful, natural healing benefits for several health conditions, including:

❀ Migraines

❀ Diarrhea

❀ Blurred vision

❀ Obesity

❀ Arthritis

❀ Stroke

❀ High blood pressure

❀ Cancer

How to Use:

Preparation:

❖ Boil cassava leaves along with sliced ginger in water for 15 minutes.

Consumption:

❖ Drink one cup daily to harness the natural healing properties.

Nature provides its own remedies for a healthier life.

For more information and support contact:
herbalifenaturescure@gmail.com

CHAPTER FIVE

QUICK WEIGHT GROWTH

TURKEY BERRY LEAVES (KWAHU NSUSUAA) AND WATERLEAF PLANT (BOKOBOKO) REMEDY

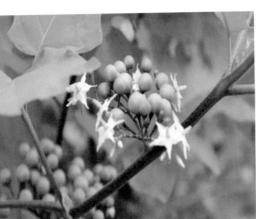

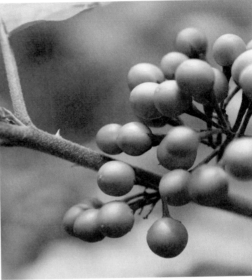

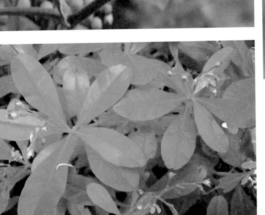

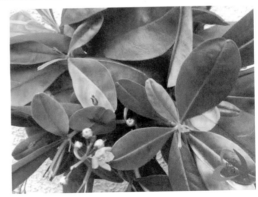

For more information and support contact:
herbalifenaturescure@gmail.com

If you're looking to increase your weight quickly, this natural remedy may help.

Instructions for Preparation:

Ingredients:

❖ Combine fresh Waterleaf plant (bokoboko) and Turkey berry (kwahu nsusuaa) leaves.

Boiling:

❖ Boil the mixture in water until well-cooked.

Usage:

❖ Drink half a glass of this remedy each morning and afternoon before meals to promote rapid weight gain.

Important Note:

Ensure that you have sufficient food available when using this remedy. Taking it without proper nutrition could be harmful to your health.

Nature provides a safe path to healthy weight gain, but proper nourishment is essential.

For more information and support contact:
herbalifenaturescure@gmail.com

CHAPTER SIX

SOURSOP LEAVES REMEDIES

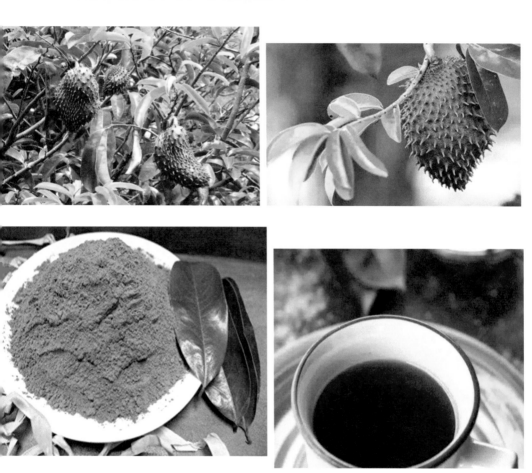

For more information and support contact:
herbalifenaturescure@gmail.com

Soursop leaves offer healing for:

🌿 Breast cancer

🌿 Prostate cancer

🌿 Blood cancer

🌿 Diabetes

🌿 Hypertension

They also help with:

🌿 Cancer

🌿 Depression

🌿 Asthma

🌿 UTI

🌿 Anaemia

🌿 High cholesterol

🌿 High blood pressure

🌿 Stomach ulcers

🌿 Menstrual pain

Illustration

- ❖ Dry the leaves,
- ❖ Grind them into a powder,
- ❖ And mix 2 tablespoons with hot water.
- ❖ Drink as tea once a day.

For more information and support contact:
herbalifenaturescure@gmail.com

CHAPTER SEVEN

CORN SILK REMEDIES

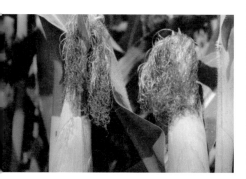

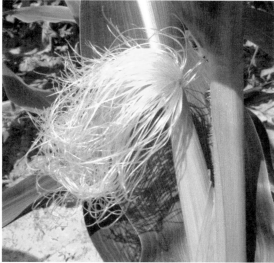

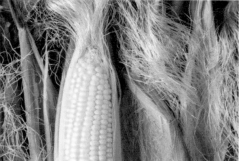

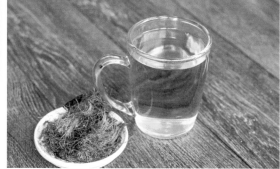

19

For more information and support contact:
herbalifenaturescure@gmail.com

Soursop Leaves: A Natural Remedy for Various Health Conditions

Soursop leaves provide healing benefits for several serious ailments, including:

🌿 Breast cancer

🌿 Prostate cancer

🌿 Blood cancer

🌿 Diabetes

🌿 Hypertension (high blood pressure)

Additionally, they can help with:

🌿 Depression

🌿 Asthma

🌿 Urinary tract infections (UTI)

🌿 Anemia

🌿 High cholesterol

🌿 Stomach ulcers

🌿 Menstrual pain

For more information and support contact:
herbalifenaturescure@gmail.com

How to Use:

Preparation:

- ❖ Dry the soursop leaves.

- ❖ Grind them into a fine powder.

Usage:

- ❖ Mix 2 tablespoons of the powder with hot water.

- ❖ Drink as tea once a day to enjoy its healing properties.

Nature offers powerful remedies for a wide range of health concerns.

For more information and support contact:
herbalifenaturescure@gmail.com

CHAPTER EIGHT

SKIN TAGS AND WARTS REMOVER

PENCIL PLANT REMEDY

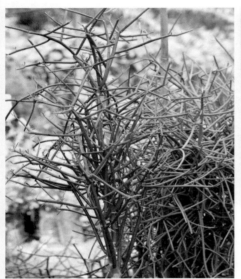
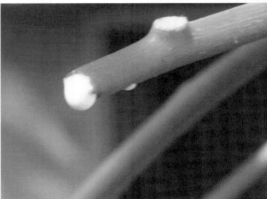
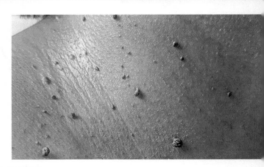
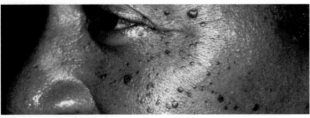

For more information and support contact:
herbalifenaturescure@gmail.com

The pencil plant is an effective natural remedy for the removal of skin tags and warts.

How to Use:

Preparation:

- ❖ Break the stem of the pencil plant to access its latex (milky sap).

Application:

- ❖ Apply the latex directly to the affected area (skin tag or wart).

Frequency:

- ❖ Repeat the process daily for one week until the skin tag falls off or the wart heals.

Nature's gentle remedy helps restore healthy skin.

For more information and support contact:
herbalifenaturescure@gmail.com

CHAPTER NINE

SICKLE CELL (SS) PATIENTS

INDIAN ALMOND PLANT REMEDY

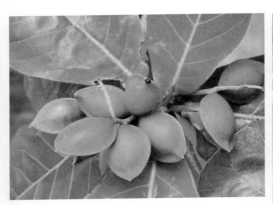
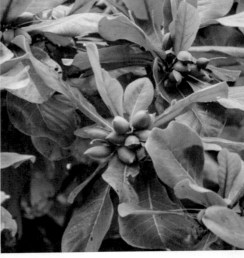
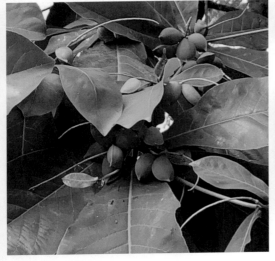
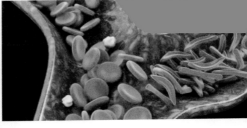

For more information and support contact:
herbalifenaturescure@gmail.com

Indian Almond Plant: A Powerful Aid for Sickle Cell (SS) Patients

The Indian almond plant offers significant benefits for individuals with Sickle Cell Disease (SS). Its strong antisickling properties help:

- ❖ Prevent frequent sickle cell crises

- ❖ Reduce the risk of anemia

- ❖ Improve blood circulation

- ❖ Alleviate pain associated with the condition

How to Use:

Preparation:

- ❖ Dry the Indian almond leaves and grind them into a powder.

Dosage:

- ❖ Take two tablespoons of the powdered leaves and brew them as tea.

Incorporating this tea into your routine can help manage the symptoms of Sickle Cell Disease, offering relief and promoting better health.

For more information and support contact:
herbalifenaturescure@gmail.com

CHAPTER TEN

PROMOTING FERTILITY IN WOMEN

AIDAN FRUIT REMEDY

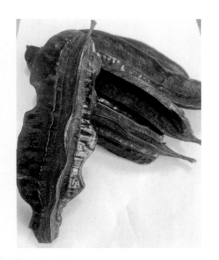

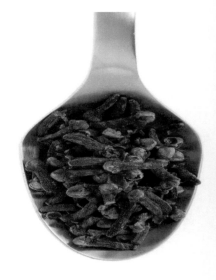

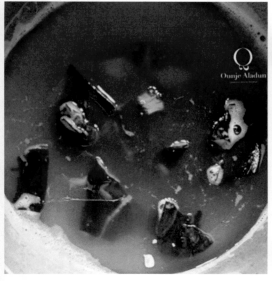

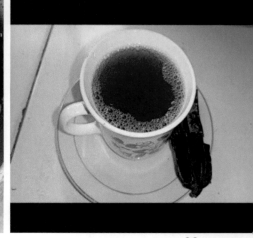

For more information and support contact:
herbalifenaturescure@gmail.com

Aidan Fruit (Prekese, Obogolo, Aridan): A Natural Boost for Women's Fertility

Aidan fruit is one of the most effective natural remedies for promoting fertility in women.

How to Use:

Preparation:

❖ Soak 3 Aidan fruits and 1 tablespoon of cloves in water overnight.

Boiling:

❖ The next day, boil the mixture for 15 minutes.

Consumption:

❖ Drink one cup daily for a month to support fertility.

Nature's remedy works wonders, wishing you a joyful and hopeful #Mother'sDay.

27

For more information and support contact:
herbalifenaturescure@gmail.com

CHAPTER ELEVEN

MALE CONTRACEPTIVE

PAWPAW/PAPAYE SEEDS REMEDY

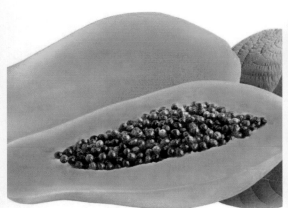
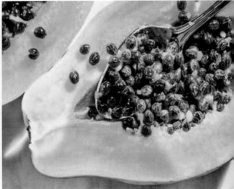

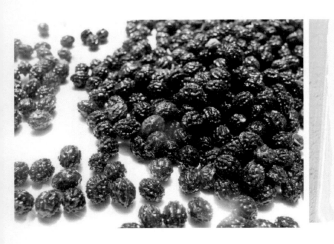
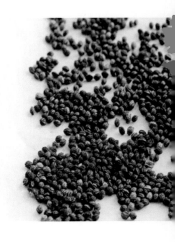

For more information and support contact:
herbalifenaturescure@gmail.com

Pawpaw Seeds: A Natural Male Contraceptive

Pawpaw seeds serve as an effective natural contraceptive for men.

How to Use:

Dosage:

Consume two tablespoons of dried Pawpaw seeds in one day.

Preparation:

Mix the seeds with hot water for consumption.

Duration of Effect:

This method can render a man sterile for up to 90 days.

Using Pawpaw seeds in this way can be a natural alternative for male contraception.

For more information and support contact:
herbalifenaturescure@gmail.com

CHAPTER TWELVE

CINNAMON, GINGER, AND TURMERIC POWDER REMEDIES

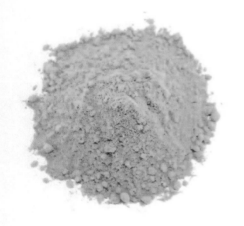
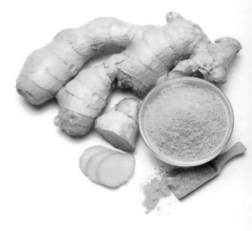

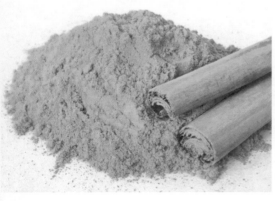
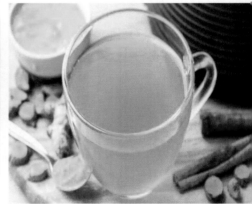

30

For more information and support contact:
herbalifenaturescure@gmail.com

A tea made from cinnamon, ginger, and turmeric powder provides relief for several health issues, including:

🌿 Colds

🌿 Kidney stones

🌿 Candidiasis (yeast infections)

🌿 Asthma

🌿 Arthritis

🌿 Waist pain

🌿 Low immunity

🌿 Hypertension (high blood pressure)

🌿 Menstrual pain

🌿 Depression

How to Prepare:

Ingredients:

- ❖ Mix 1 teaspoon of cinnamon powder, 1 teaspoon of ginger powder, and 1 teaspoon of turmeric powder.

Preparation:

- ❖ Add the mixture to hot water.

Consumption:

- ❖ Drink this tea first thing in the morning to experience its health benefits.

Embrace nature's healing touch with this powerful herbal tea!

For more information and support contact:
herbalifenaturescure@gmail.com

CHAPTER THIRTEEN

VARIOUS CANCERS

MANGO PEELS REMEDIES

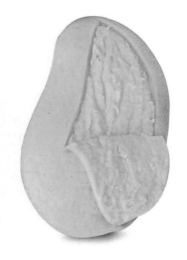
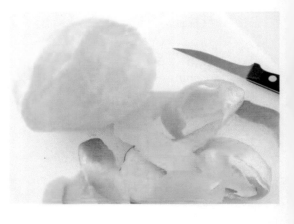
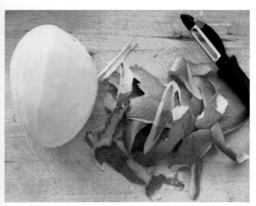
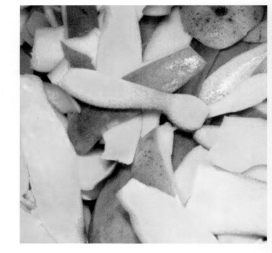

For more information and support contact:
herbalifenaturescure@gmail.com

Mango peels are highly effective in both preventing and treating various types of cancer, including:

❈ Colon cancer

❈ Lung cancer

❈ Prostate cancer

❈ Cervical cancer

In addition to their anticancer benefits, mango peels also provide relief for several other health conditions, such as:

❈ Arthritis

❈ Stomach ulcers

❈ The common cold

❈ Diabetes

How to Use:

Consumption Methods:

❖ *Chewing:* You can chew the mango pulp along with the peel for maximum benefit.

Boiling:

❖ Alternatively, boil the peel in water and drink the resulting liquid.

Nature offers powerful healing benefits through mango peels, making them a valuable addition to your health regimen.

For more information and support contact:
herbalifenaturescure@gmail.com

CHAPTER FOURTEEN

GINGER, CLOVES, AND GARLIC REMEDIES

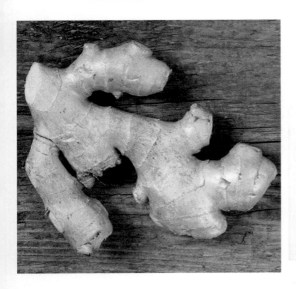
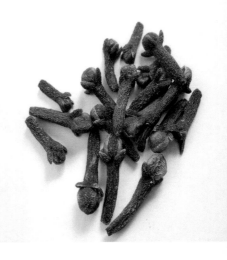
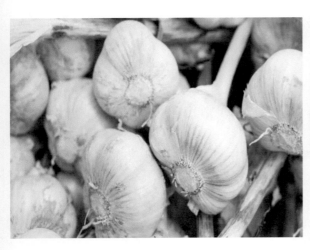
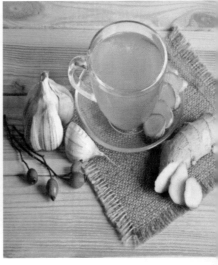

For more information and support contact:
herbalifenaturescure@gmail.com

Drinking tea made from ginger, cloves, and garlic is an effective remedy for several health issues, including:

❊ Urinary tract infections

❊ Hypertension (high blood pressure)

❊ Cough

❊ Arthritis

❊ High cholesterol

❊ Low immunity

❊ Painful menstruation

❊ Gonorrhea

How to Prepare:

Ingredients:

- ❖ Ginger, cloves, and garlic.

Preparation:

- ❖ Grind or chop the ingredients into smaller pieces.

- ❖ Boil them in water for 15 minutes.

Consumption:

- ❖ Drink one teacup of the tea twice daily to experience optimal health benefits.

This natural remedy harnesses the powerful properties of ginger, cloves, and garlic to support overall wellness.

35

For more information and support contact:
herbalifenaturescure@gmail.com

CHAPTER FIFTEEN

AVOCADO (PEAR) SEED REMEDY

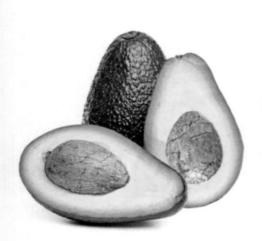
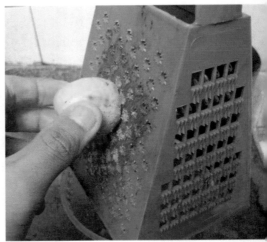

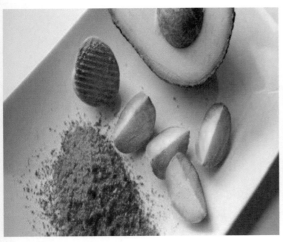
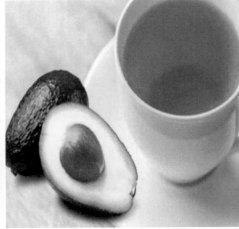

For more information and support contact:
herbalifenaturescure@gmail.com

Avocado Seeds: A Natural Remedy for Various Health Conditions

Avocado (pear) seeds are effective in treating several health issues, including:

❄ High blood pressure

❄ High cholesterol

❄ Asthma

❄ Low immunity

❄ Blood cancer

❄ Obesity

❄ Candidiasis (yeast infections)

How to Use:

Preparation:

- ❖ *Grating:* Grate the avocado seeds and add them to smoothies, salads, or soups for an easy way to incorporate them into your diet.

Alternative Method:

- ❖ *Powdering:* Alternatively, grind the seeds into a fine powder.

- ❖ *Mixing:* Mix two tablespoons of the powdered seed with hot water.

Consumption:

- ❖ Drink the mixture once daily to enjoy the health benefits.

Incorporating avocado seeds into your diet can support overall health and well-being.

For more information and support contact:
herbalifenaturescure@gmail.com

CHAPTER SIXTEEN

MOUTH ULCERS OR CANKER SORES

CLOVES REMEDIES

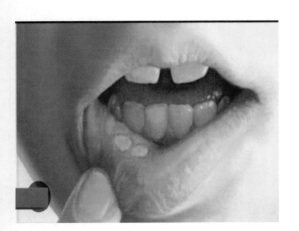 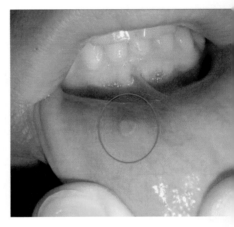

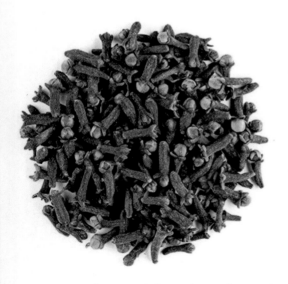 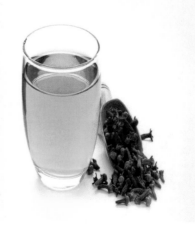

For more information and support contact:
herbalifenaturescure@gmail.com

Cloves are an effective remedy for treating mouth ulcers or canker sores.

How to Use:

Preparation:

❖ Boil three tablespoons of cloves in water.

Rinsing:

❖ Use the strained water to rinse your mouth both in the morning and before bed.

Important Note:

❖ Be sure to spit out the water after rinsing.

This natural remedy promotes healing, showcasing the power of nature in supporting oral health.

For more information and support contact:
herbalifenaturescure@gmail.com

CHAPTER SEVENTEEN

THE MAST TREE REMEDIES

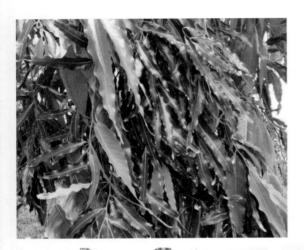
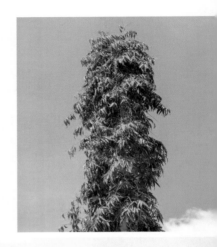
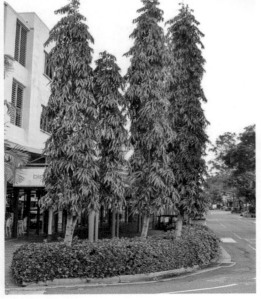
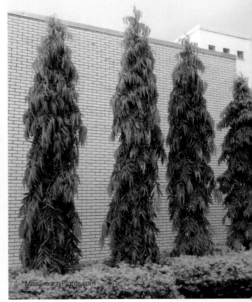

For more information and support contact:
herbalifenaturescure@gmail.com

Mast Tree: A Natural Remedy for Various Health Conditions

The mast tree is known for its healing properties, effectively addressing a variety of ailments, including:

- ❈ Malaria
- ❈ Typhoid fever
- ❈ Candidiasis (yeast infections)
- ❈ Arthritis
- ❈ Stomach ulcers
- ❈ Hypertension (high blood pressure)
- ❈ Diabetes
- ❈ Liver dysfunction
- ❈ Intestinal worm infestations

How to Use:

Preparation:

- ❖ Boil three tablespoons of dried, powdered leaves in water for 10 minutes.

Consumption:

- ❖ Drink one teacup of the strained mixture twice daily for optimal results.

This natural remedy harnesses the power of the mast tree to promote healing and improve overall health.

For more information and support contact:
herbalifenaturescure@gmail.com

Thanks for joining us to celebrate the launch of The Holistic Guide to Wellness: Herbal Remedies for Common Ailments!

I'm so grateful to everyone for being here with us today! It really means a lot to have you here!

Dear readers,

I really appreciate your support and interest in The Holistic Guide to Wellness: Herbal Remedies for Common Ailments. Thanks a bunch! This book is a wonderful resource for tapping into the natural healing abilities of plants to address a variety of health issues, such as rheumatism, obesity, typhoid fever, hypertension, blood cancer, diabetes, stomach ulcers, hepatitis, and many others.

It's wonderful to see your enthusiasm for exploring herbal remedies, showcasing your dedication to well-being and a holistic approach to health. I would love it if you could take a moment to share your thoughts by writing a review of the book. Your feedback means so much to us! It really helps us improve and supports other readers in making informed health choices.

Also, it would be great to share this wonderful resource with students, parents, friends, and medical professionals! This information can assist others in understanding and appreciating natural healing, fostering a greater awareness of the healing power of plants.

Thanks a bunch for your purchase! Let's set off on this adventure to discover the amazing healing power of nature together!

Warm regards,

For more information and support contact:
herbalifenaturescure@gmail.com

Made in the USA
Columbia, SC
09 December 2024

48885705R00024